Stay Fit and Healthy with the Mediterranean Diet

Simple, tasty recipes to brighten your daily meals

Lana Green

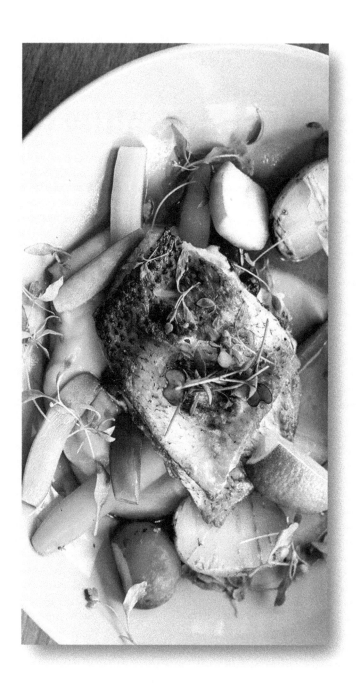

Table of Contents

Pecorino pasta with sausage and tomato

Prep Time: 20 min

Cook Time: 20 min

Serve: 4

Ingredients:

- 2 tsp olive oil

- 1 cup sliced onion

- 8 oz penne

- 8 oz Italian sausage

- 6 tbsp grated Romano cheese

- 1/4 tsp salt

- 2 tsp garlic

- 1 1/4 lb tomatoes

- 1/8 tsp black pepper

- 1/4 cup torn basil leaves

Preparation:

1. Boil & drain pasta. Keep the boiled pasta aside.

2. Now at a full flame, heat a skillet, which should be nonstick. Take oil in a pan & add sausage and onion to it.

3. Cook for about two minutes. Now remove from stove & add pasta, salt, black pepper powder & cheese. Add oil to a pan, swirl to coat. Sprinkle remaining 1/4th cup of cheese and serve.

Pesto pasta and shrimp

Prep Time: 10 min

Cook Time: 10 min

Serve: 3

Ingredients:

- 10 oz spaghetti

- 3/4 cup basil pesto

- 1 lb shrimp

- 1 tbsp olive oil

- 1 tsp Italian seasoning

- Salt to taste

- Black pepper to taste

- 1/4 cup parmesan cheese

Preparation:

1. Bring a pot of salted water to a boil and cook the pasta While the pasta is cooking, prepare the shrimp. Heat the olive oil in a pan over high heat.

2. Add the shrimp and sprinkle with Italian seasoning, salt and pepper. Cook for 2-4 minutes or until shrimp is just pink and opaque. Turn off the heat.

3. Drain the pasta and add it to the pan with the shrimp. Stir in the pesto. Add the cherry tomatoes and parmesan cheese to the pan. Garnish with parsley if desired.

Spanish rice casserole with cheesy beef

Prep Time: 10 min

Cook Time: 25 min

Serve: 4

Ingredients:

- 16.8 oz Spanish Rice mix

- 1 tbsp olive oil

- One red bell pepper

- 1 cup of corn

- 1 cup meatless crumbles

- 1/3 cup sour cream

- 1/4 cup salsa

- 1/2 cup Monterey Jack cheese

- 2 tbsp crumbled queso fresco

- One avocado sliced

Preparation:

1. Prepare the rice in a 2.5-liter casserole dish, which should be microwavable. Preheat the microwave up to 375 F.

2. Take a skillet and heat the oil. Now cook bell pepper till tendered 5-7 minutes. Once the rice is cooked, then combine the bell pepper, cooked, meatless crumbles, salsa, sour cream & corn. Now sprinkle the cheese on the top.

3. Bake it, uncovered (10 minutes), till the cheese is melted & browned on top. Top sliced avocado.

Yangchow Chinese style fried rice

Prep Time: 15 min

Cook Time: 20 min

Serve: 6

Ingredients:

- 6 cups cooked white rice

- 1 cup barbecued pork

- 1 tsp sugars

- 1 tsp ginger

- Ten pieces of shrimps

- 3/4 cup green peas

- 1 tsp garlic

- 1 1/2 tbsp soy sauce

- 2 tsp salt

- 1/4 cup green onion

- Two beaten eggs

- 3 tbsp cooking oil

Preparation:

1. Heat the oil & sauté ginger-garlic together. Add the shrimps & cook (1 minute). Pour the egg mixture & cook.

2. Divide the cooked egg into pieces. Add rice & soy sauce, salt & sugar, and mix with other ingredients.

3. Add pork, which is barbecued & cook (3 minutes). Add peas & shrimp & cook 3 minutes. Add onions and cook (2 minutes). Turn off heat & transfer to a serving plate.

Mahi-mahi pomegranate sauce

Prep Time: 5 min

Cook Time: 20 min

Serve: 2

Ingredients:

- 12 oz Mahi-mahi fillets
- 1/2 cup balsamic vinegar
- 1/4 cup pomegranate juice
- 1 tbsp olive oil
- 1 tbsp squeezed lemon juice
- 1/2 cup pomegranate seeds

Preparation:

1. Preheat microwave up to 450 deg. Take baking dish & lay

Mahi fillets, drizzle with lemon juice & olive oil.

2. Bake it for 15-20 minutes Take a pan & heat vinegar pomegranate juice & seeds over high heat.

3. Bring a boil & let the sauce to reduce (20 minutes). Spoon the fillets. Serve & enjoy.

Feta tomato sea bass

Prep Time: 10 min

Cook Time: 10 min

Serve: 4

Ingredients:

- 2 oz dry white wine

- 2 tbsp lemon juice

- 32 oz sea bass fillets

- 4 oz feta cheese

- Five ripe tomatoes

- 5 tbsp olive oil

- 2 tbsp butter

- 2 tbsp basil

- Three garlic cloves

- 1 tbsp oregano

- Salt & pepper

Preparation:

1. Take fish & rub salt & pepper over it. Heat the pan & add olive oil. Put the fish in a pan.

2. Cook it until it is golden brown. Add basil, cheese, lemon juice, tomatoes & garlic. Bake 12-15 minutes at 400 deg. Take the dish out and finish it with butter.

3. The dish is ready. Now serve and enjoy.

Crab stew

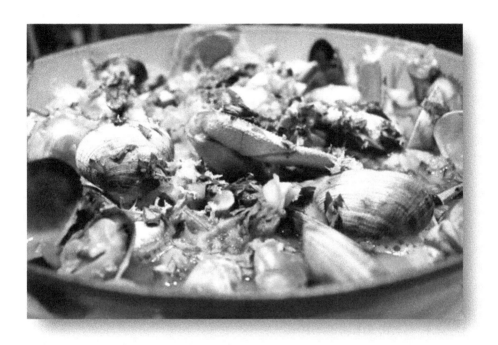

Prep Time: 25 min

Cook Time: 25 min

Serve: 4

Ingredients:

- 2 tbsp sweet paprika
- 1/2 cup heavy cream

- 6 tbsp unsalted butter

- 1/4 lb shrimp

- 1 lb lump crabmeat

- 2 cups steamed rice

- 3/4 tsp chipotle Chile powder

- 2 tbsp all-purpose flour

- 1/4 cup dry sherry

- 2 cups clam juice

- 1 cup of water

- One small onion

- One garlic clove

- Salt and pepper

- 1 tbsp leaf parsley

Preparation:

1. Melt one tbsp of butter in a pan. Add shrimp & cook at moderate heat. Now add sherry & cook for 2 minutes.

2. Add clam juice & water. Bring a boil & simmer moderately at low heat for 10 minutes. Strain broth. Now again, melt 2 tbsp butter in the pan. Add garlic & onion & cook at moderate heat till it is softened. Add paprika & chipotle, stirring for 3 minutes. Now stir with flour. Whisk broth in the pan. Cook till it becomes smooth & then bring a boil. Simmer at low heat. Whisk till it is just thickened 5 minutes. Add cream, simmer & season with salt & pepper.

3. Take a skillet & melt 3 tbsp butter. Now gently stir the crab & cook at moderate heat. Toss for a few minutes' till warmed 4 minutes. Season with salt & pepper, Spoon steamed rice into the shallow bowls, Ladle shellfish sauce on rice & top with crab. Sprinkle with parsley & serve.

Savory zucchini loaf

Prep Time: 25 min

Cook time: 50-55 min

Serve: 8

Ingredients:

- 5 tbsp of olive oil

- One small, diced zucchini.

- Half cup of hazelnuts.

- ¾ cup of tomato (sun-dried).

- Half cup milk

- One cup all-purpose flour

- Three eggs

- 2 tsp of baking powder

- 2/3 cup of mozzarella cheese.

- ¼ cup of basil.

- ¼ tbsp of black pepper

- ¼ tbsp of sea salt

Preparation:

1. Preheat the microwave up to 350 F Toast hazelnuts on moderate heat in a frypan. Sauté diced zucchini on medium heat (5 min). Place tomatoes in a bowl. For ten minutes, cover it with hot water. Drain it and place it aside.

2. Take three eggs and whisk them in a bowl. Add milk to eggs & beat. Add flour & baking soda mix until it becomes smooth. Add 5 tbsp of olive oil & pepper. Mix it well.

3. Add other ingredients tomatoes, basil, hazelnuts & mozzarella. Mix delicately with a spatula. Spray the pan with cooking spray & pour the batter into it. Bake for almost 45 min until toothpick comes out dry and clean. Cut it into slices & serve.

Chilled Pea and mint soup

Prep Time: 20 min

Cook Time: 20-25 min

Serve: 4

Ingredients:

- 2 tbsp of butter

- One chopped onion medium size.

- Two cups of water

- Two pounds of frozen green peas

- Two cups of vegetable broth.

- ¼ cup of fresh mint leaves

- ¼ cup of fresh parsley

- 1 tsp of fresh lemon juice

- Half tsp cayenne

- Mint leaves for garnishing

Preparation:

1. Melt the butter in a large pan. Add onions & cook till softened for 7 minutes. Combine vegetable stock & water in a medium-sized saucepan.

2. Stir in 1/2 of the water mixture in the large pan along with the onions. Increase the heat & bring to boil. Add peas & bring to a boil for one minute. Remove from stove.

3. Add remaining water mixture with the mint, parsley & cayenne. Puree with an immersion blender in a pot till it becomes smooth. Season using lime juice.

4. Cool until chilled. Serve in the bowls with mint leaves.

Watermelon & cantaloupe salad

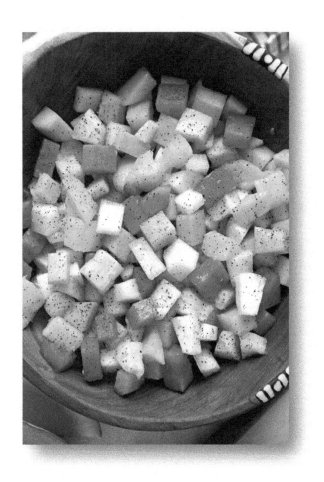

Prep Time: 10 min

Cook Time: 0 min

Serve: 6

Ingredients:

- ¼ cup of pine nuts

- 2 cups of diced cantaloupe

- Six cups of diced watermelon

- 5 tbsp of olive oil

- 2/3 cup of crumbled feta cheese

- 1/4 cup of fresh mint.

- ¼ tsp of black pepper powder

Preparation:

1. Toast pine nuts in a pan. Add olive oil, cantaloupe & watermelon in a bowl. Sprinkle the cheese, mint & pepper.

2. Mix it delicately. Chill for one hour. Serve.

Southern-fried okra

Prep Time: 5 min

Cook Time: 25 min

Serve: 6

Ingredients:

- Half cup flour-unbleached
- Half cup of cornmeal.
- 1/8th tsp of salt
- 1/4th tsp of fresh black pepper
- One egg
- Two tbsp of milk
- 1/3rd cup of sunflower oil
- 3 cups of fresh okra

Preparation:

1. Preheat the microwave up to 300 F. Mix & whisk together the flour, salt, black pepper & cayenne in a bowl.

2. Beat egg & milk in a bowl. Heat sunflower oil.

3. Dip okra pieces in the egg batter & roll in a mixture.

4. Fry in the pan. Turn over after two min. Remove the cooked okra with a spoon & drain each batch. Transfer 1st batch to a baking dish to keep it warm while the remaining okra is cooking.

5. Place the 2nd batch of the fried okra in the oven till the final batch is done. Serve it immediately.

Pesto Pasta with Peas and Mozzarella

Prep Time: 10 min

Cook Time: 0 min

Serve: 3

Ingredients:

- 2 cups green peas

- 1 cup mozzarella balls low sodium

- 4 cups Boiled Penna Pasta

- 2 cups fresh basil leaves

- ¼ tsp Garlic powder

- 1 tbsp Lemon juice

- 2 tsp zest of a lemon

- 1/3 cup olive oil

- ¼ tsp Salt

- ¼ tsp Pepper

Preparation:

1. For making pesto, add all the ingredients in a blender or food processor and mix them except for olive oil. Pulse until crudely sliced. Reduce the food processor's speed or blender, slowly add olive oil to it, mix it well, and blend.

2. Scrape down the sides of the food processor/blender to fully mix the end. Add salt & pepper.

3. Add mozzarella, pasta, and peas into a large bowl. Add pesto according to requirement Add pesto as desired and then mix all ingredients.

Balsamic Roasted Green Beans

Prep Time: 5 min

Cook Time: 17 min

Serve: 1 cup

Ingredients:

- 1 lb Green beans
- 2 Chopped Garlic Cloves
- 1 tbsp Balsamic vinegar
- 1 tbsp Olive oil
- ⅛ tsp Salt
- ⅛ tsp Pepper

Preparation:

1. Preheat oven to 425°F. Mix green beans along with olive oils, pepper & salt in a large bowl.

2. Evenly spread green beans on a foil or parchment paper-lined on a baking sheet. Bake them for 10-12 mints in the oven until it turns light brown.

3. Spread garlic with green beans & mix well to combine. Then again, bake it for another 5 minutes till beans are warm & browned.

4. Remove from oven & toss with balsamic vinegar.

Mac in a Flash (Macaroni and Cheese)

Prep Time: 2 min

Cook Time: 10 min

Serve: 4

Ingredients:

- 3 cups Water
- 1 cup Noodles
- ½ cup Grated Cheddar Cheese
- 1 tsp Butter
- ⅛ tsp dry mustard

Preparation:

1. Add noodles in boiling water, boil it for 5 to 7 minutes or until tender, and then drain the boiled noodles.

2. Sprinkle the grated cheddar cheese on the hot noodles & mix it with butter and dry grounded mustard.

Costa Rican Gallo Pinto

Prep Time: 5 min

Cook Time: 30 min

Serve: 4

Ingredients:

- 1/3 cup dry black beans

- 4 tbsp Olive oil

- 110g Chopped Onion

- 2 Chopped Garlic Cloves

- One chopped red bell pepper

- 1 tsp Cumin

- 1 tbsp Salsa Lizano

- 3 cups Cooked White rice

- ½ tsp black pepper

- Bit of smoked paprika

- ¼ cup Chopped Cilantro

- 4 Hard-boiled eggs
- Salt to taste

Preparation:

Preparation of beans advance:

1. Soak black beans in one and a half cups of water at least for 2 hrs. or overnight.

2. Add beans in boiling water and boil them until beans tender for ten- fifteen. Save beans along with water.

Preparation for Gallo pinto:

1. Take a large frying pan and heat the oil over medium heat.

2. Then add sliced veggies (garlic, onion, & red pepper) to it.

3. Fry and stir it while frying unless or until vegies becomes soft & aromatic. After adding cumin and salsa Lozano in it, mix, then gin cook gin for two to three more minutes.

4. Now mix the boiled bens and its water in it and again cook for just one mint. Combine the cooked rice & make sure that stir until rice is completely mixed with the beans.

5. Cover the frying pan, reduce the heat & cook again for one to two minutes, till the rice is warmed. Flavor with smoked paprika, pepper & cilantro for good flavor.

6. Finally, add this to a bowl and decorate it with a hard-boiled egg on top.

Cheese Quiche

Prep Time: 5 min

Cook Time: 45 min

Serve: 8

Ingredients:

- 4 Marginally beaten eggs
- Splash of Pepper
- 1.5 cup milk
- 3 oz shredded cheddar cheese
- ¼ cup Chopped onion
- 1 tsp Parsley leaves
- Pastry shell un-baked

Preparation:

1. Preheat oven to 350°F. Mix all ingredients in a large bowl & mix it perfectly.

2. Now add already prepared unbaked pastry shell. Bake this for forty to forty-five minutes.

3. Cut into eight slices but cool this before baking.

Cheesy thyme waffles

Prep Time: 10 min

Cook Time: 7 min

Serve: 2

Ingredients:

- Two eggs

- 1/3 cup parmesan cheese

- 1 tsp garlic powder

- 1 tsp thyme

- 1 cup collard greens

- 1 tbsp olive oil

- Two stalks onion

- 1/2 cauliflower

- 1/2 tsp salt

- 1 cup shredded mozzarella cheese

- 1 tbsp of sesame seeds

- 1/2 tsp black pepper

Preparation:

1. Cut cauliflower & slice onions. Add cauliflower to the blender. Add onions, thyme & collard greens to the blender & pulse again. Now add the processed mixture to a bowl.

2. Mix it well to form a smooth batter. A heat waffle iron.

3. Pour the mixture into the waffle iron, ensuring that it is spread properly. Cook well & serve hot.

Baked egg and asparagus with cheese parmesan

Prep Time: 10 min

Cook Time: 15 min

Serve: 3

Ingredients:

- 30 spears asparagus
- Six eggs
- 3 tbsp parmesan cheese
- 3/4 tsp salt
- 3 tsp butter
- 3 tsp olive oil
- 3/4 tsp black pepper

Preparation:

1. Preheat microwave up to 400 deg. Take a small pot of water. Add salt & add asparagus. Stir it well.

2. When water boils again, please remove it from the stove.

3. Drain asparagus & transfer it to a bowl filled with cold water. Distribute asparagus.

4. Among three baking dishes, Top center of the baking dish along with one tsp of butter. Season with salt.

5. Add eggs to the baking dish. Bake for 10 min. Remove it from the microwave. Top each portion with cheese & black pepper. Return to microwave & bake it for 7 min.

6. Serve and enjoy.

Creamy cold salad

Prep Time: 10 min

Cook Time: 1 min

Serve: 3

Ingredients:

- 8 oz salad macaroni
- 1/4 sliced green onion
- 1/2 cup red pepper
- 1/2 cup black olives
- 1 cup broccoli florets
- 1/2 cup cucumber

Dressing:

- 1/2 cup mayonnaise
- 2 tsp vinegar
- 1/2 tsp kosher salt

- 1/2 tsp black pepper

- 1/2 tsp sugar

Preparation:

1. Cook pasta. When noodles are cooked, add broccoli.

2. Let broccoli boil 40 sec. Drain everything. Rinse well

3. Stir with mayonnaise, salt, pepper, vinegar & sugar in a

bowl. Add cooked pasta & broccoli in a bowl & stir well.

4. Add cucumber, olives, pepper, & onion. Stir again.

5. Cover & refrigerate until the ready dish is ready to serve.

6. Stir again before serving. Enjoy the food!

Peppy pepper tomato salad

Prep Time: 5 min

Cook Time: 10 min

Serve: 4

Ingredients:

- One small garlic
- 1/4 cup olive oil
- 1 tbsp sherry vinegar
- 1 tsp balsamic vinegar
- Salt and pepper
- 1 pound tomatoes
- 1.5 pounds red peppers
- 1 tbsp basil
- One leaf lettuce

Preparation:

1. Mix sherry vinegar, garlic, olive oil, balsamic vinegar, salt, and black pepper powder according to taste. Cut roasted peppers strips. Toss with dressing.

2. Add 1/2 basil & toss again. Remove & discard tough outer leaves. Wash & dry the leaves & tear them to pieces.

3. Toss with tomatoes & dressing & basil. Line platter. Top with peppers. Serve slightly chilled.

Spinach and grilled feta salad

Prep Time: 10 min

Cook Time: 20 min

Serve: 1

Ingredients:

- 1/2 tbsp olive oil

- 1 oz feta cheese

- 1 cup shredded mozzarella cheese

- One pinch of salt

- pepper to taste

- One clove garlic

- Two ciabatta rolls

- 1/4 lb spinach

Preparation:

1. Mince garlic & add to a pan with olive oil. Cook at moderate heat for 3 minutes. Add frozen spinach & turn heat up. Cook 5 minutes. Season it lightly with sea salt & black pepper. Cut rolls in half.

2. Add shredded mozzarella & half oz. of feta to bottom. Divide cooked spinach. Then top each sandwich with a pinch of red pepper plus more mozzarella. Place top of ciabatta roll on sandwiches & transfer in a non- stick pan

3. Fill the pot with water for creating weight. Place pot on the top of sandwiches to press them. Flip sandwiches carefully. Place the weighted pot on top & cook. Serve hot and enjoy.

Salmon and Cucumber Salad

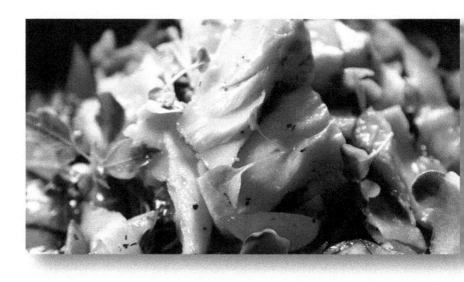

Prep Time: 8 min

Cook Time: 35 min

Serve: 4

Ingredients:

- Sauce

- 1/4 tsp kosher salt

- 2 tsp lemon juice

- 13 tsp pepper

- 1 tbsp olive oil

- 1 tbsp chopped dill

- 1 cup yogurt

- Cucumber salad

- 2 tsp olive oil

- 2 tsp chopped flat-leaf parsley

- 2 tsp chopped chives

- 13 tsp pepper

- 13 tsp kosher salt

- 1.5 tsp minced shallot

- ¾ tsp lemon juice

- ½ lb English cucumbers

- Salmon and serving

- ¼ tsp kosher salt

- ¼ tsp pepper

- 1 tbsp olive oil

- Four salmon fillets

- Dill sprigs

Preparation:

1. Mix all the ingredients of the sauce list in a bowl. The sauce is ready. Combine all the items of salad in a bowl and set aside. The salad and dressing are ready.

2. Place fish with skin placed downwards on a baking tray.

3. Grill the fillets for 15 minutes. Place the grilled fillets on a plate and drizzle salad and dressing over it; serve.

Salmon, Lentil & Pomegranate Salad

Prep Time: 15 min

Cook Time: 0 min

Serve: 2

Ingredients:

- One garlic clove chopped

- One red onion sliced

- 1 tsp clear honey

- One pomegranate

- 140 g hot-smoked salmon

- 2 tbsp olive oil

- 2 tbsp chopped tarragon

- 20 g flat-leaf parsley

- 400 g lentil

- juice ½ lemon

- toasted pitta bread, to serve

Preparation:

Combine all the ingredients in a bowl and toss well. Serve

and enjoy it.

Salmon and pumpkin salad with chili jam

Prep Time: 30 min

Cook Time: 30 min

Serve: 2

Ingredients:

- lime

- coriander (chopped to serve)

- 700 g pumpkin

- Four salmon fillets

- 200 g green beans

- 125 g baby spinach

- 1 tbsp olive oil

- One sliced Spanish onion

Dressing:

- 2 tbsp lime juice

- 1/2 cup vegetable stock (liquid)

- 1 tbsp fish sauce

- 1 tbsp chili jam

- 1 tbsp brown sugar

Preparation:

1. Combine all the items of dressing in a pan and boil it for few minutes. The dressing is ready. Drizzle oil over pumpkin and roast in a preheated oven at 200 degrees for 25 minutes.

2. Add peas to boiling water and cook for five minutes. Cook salmon in a heated pan for five minutes. Now mix all the items in a bowl and pour dressing.

Salmon with Pomegranate Molasses Glaze

Prep Time: 5 min

Cook Time: 15 min

Serve: 3

Ingredients:

- 1/2 tsp salt

- 1/4 cup pomegranate molasses

- 1/4 tsp cornstarch

- 2 tsp brown sugar

- Four boneless salmon fillets

- Black pepper

- pomegranate seeds for garnish

- Mint for garnishing

Preparation:

1. Whisk pepper, sugar, salt, and starch in a bowl. Coat fillets with the mixture.

2. Fry the fillets in heated oil for five minutes. Transfer the fillets to the baking tray. Drizzle pomegranate molasses over fillets.

3. Bake in a preheated oven at 400 degrees for 15 minutes.

Scallops and Summer Vegetable Skillet

Prep Time: 15 min

Cook Time: 15 min

Serve: Adjustable

Ingredients:

- 1/2 cup diced zucchini

- 1 cup corn kernels

- One sliced cherry tomatoes

- 1 lb scallops

- 1 tbsp olive oil

- Three cloves garlic minced

- 3 tbsp diced shallots

- 3 tbsp salted butter

- Salt to taste pepper to taste

Preparation:

1. Cook scallops in a heated oven over medium flame for three minutes. Transfer it to a plate. Sauté shallots and garlic in the same pan over medium flame. Stir in zucchini and tomatoes for ten minutes.

2. Mix in corn, salt, and black pepper. Add scallop and cook for five minutes.

Tuna Patties

Prep Time: 15 min

Cook Time: 10 min

Serve: 4

Ingredients:

- 3 tbsp vegetable oil

- 3 tbsp grated Parmesan cheese

- 3 tbsp diced Onion

- 15 oz tuna

- 2 tsp lemon juice

- Two eggs

- 10 tbsp bread crumbs

- One pinch of black pepper

Preparation:

Whisk all the items in a bowl. Make patties out of the mixture. Fry the patties in heated oil over medium flame for five minutes.

Whole Salmon Fillet with Crispy Lemon & Basil Crumb Topping

Prep Time: 15 min

Cook Time: 18 min

Serve: 4

Ingredients:

- Salt to taste

- black pepper to taste

- Two cloves garlic

- 1.45 lb salmon fillet

- 1 tbsp lemon juice

- 1 tbsp lemon thyme

- 1 lb asparagus

- One lemon, zested

- 1 cup bread crumbs

- ½ tsp salt

- ½ tsp black pepper

- 1/3 cup grated Parmesan cheese

- 1/3 cup chopped fresh basil

- ¼ cup olive oil, divided

Preparation:

1. Season salmon with oil, pepper, and salt. Shift the salmon in the pan. Mix asparagus with oil and salt and place around salmon. Blend garlic, cheese, basil, thyme, lemon juice, zest, salt, and pepper in a food processor.

2. Pour the mixture over salmon. Bake in the oven for 20 minutes.

Seafood paella

Prep Time: 15 min

Cook Time: 55 min

Serve: 6

Ingredients:

- Two ¼ cups chicken broth

- 2 tsp olive oil

- 1 lb jumbo shrimp

- ½ teaspoon saffron threads

- salt to taste

- 8 oz sliced chorizo sausage

- Two cloves garlic, minced

- 1 1/3 cups Arborio rice

- 1 tsp paprika

- 1 tbsp olive oil

- One sliced red bell pepper

- One pinch of cayenne pepper

- ½ yellow onion, diced

- ½ cup green peas

Preparation:

1. Fry chorizo in heated oil for three minutes. Mix in onions and cook for three more minutes.

2. Stir in rice and peas and toss well. Place shrimp over rice and bake for twenty minutes.

Thyme-Scented Salmon with White Bean Salad

Prep Time: 15 min

Cook Time: 0 min

Serve: 4

Ingredients:

- Bean Salad

- 3 tbsp lemon juice

- 2 tsp chopped parsley

- 2 tsp chopped mint

- 2 tsp chopped basil

- 2 tbsp water

- Two garlic cloves, minced

- 1 tbsp olive oil

- 15 oz cannellini beans

- ½ cup chopped shallots

- ½ cup chopped carrot

- 1/3 cup chopped celery

- Salmon

- Four salmon fillets

- 3 tbsp lemon juice

- 2 tsp chopped thyme

- 13 tsp black pepper

- 1 tsp chopped parsley

- ½ tsp salt

Preparation:

1. Cook celery, carrot, shallots, and garlic in heated oil over medium flame for five minutes. Mix all the ingredients and cook. Place the mixture in salmon.

2. Bake salmon in a preheated oven at 375 degrees for 15 minutes.

Curry Chicken Salad

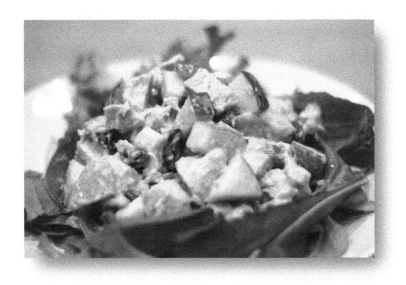

Prep Time: 15 min

Cook Time: 15 min

Serve: 6

Ingredients:

- Three cooked chicken breasts

- 2/3 cup chopped celery

- 2 tbsp lemon juice

- 1/4 tsp black pepper

- 1/4 cup sliced chives

- 1/3 cup raisins

- 1/2 tsp salt

- 1/2 cup roasted salted cashews

- 1/2 cup mayonnaise

- 1 tbsp yellow curry powder

- One tart apple

Preparation:

Whisk all the items in the bowl and serve.

Grilled Indian Chicken

Prep Time: 35 min

Cook Time: 10 min

Serve: 4

Ingredients:

- 4 boneless chicken breasts

Marinade

- 1/4 tsp cayenne pepper

- 1/2 tsp ginger

- 1/2 cup plain yogurt

- 1 tsp cumin

- 1 tsp coriander

- 1 tbsp paprika

- 1 tbsp onion powder

- 1 tbsp minced garlic

- 1 tbsp lemon juice

- 1 tbsp garam masala

- 1 tbsp cilantro leaves

Preparation:

Combine all the items in a bowl and set aside. Grill chicken over a grill for seven minutes from both sides.

Hearty Turkey Stew

Prep Time: 10 min

Cook Time: 60 min

Serve: 4

Ingredients:

- 100 g sliced bacon lardons
- 1/3 cup heavy cream
- 1 tbsp butter
- One leek
- Two sliced carrots
- Two stalks celery diced
- Two cloves garlic pressed
- 2 tbsp flour, heaped
- 4 cups chicken or turkey stock
- 2 cups cooked turkey
- Two chopped potatoes

- Two bay leaves

- 1 tbsp thyme leaves

- 1 tbsp chopped parsley

- salt to taste

- pepper to taste

Preparation:

1. Fry bacon in butter over medium flame. Stir in leeks, carrots, thyme, and celery, and cook for five minutes. Mix garlic and cook again for one minute.

2. Add flour, pepper, and salt. Mix potatoes, bay leaves, and turkey and cook for 50 minutes. Add heavy cream and serve.

Herb and Orange Chicken

Prep Time: 10 min

Cook Time: 60 min

Serve: 4

Ingredients:

- 1/4 cup ghee
- 3 1/2 oranges
- 4.5 lb chicken
- Three yellow potatoes
- Two stems of rosemary
- Six stems of thyme
- salt & pepper

Preparation:

Heat orange juice in ghee over medium flame and set aside. Place chicken, potatoes, orange slices, thyme, and rosemary. Bake for one hour and serve with orange sauce.

Pomegranate Walnut & Chicken Stew

Prep Time: 15 min

Cook Time: 75 min

Serve: 5

Ingredients:

- 1 cups California walnuts

- pinch salt

- pepper

- 2 tbsp olive oil

- 1 tbsp butter

- Four cloves garlic chopped

- 1 tsp turmeric

- 1 tsp cumin

- One cinnamon stick

- ½ tsp nutmeg

- ½ tsp black pepper orange zest

- 2 cups chicken stock

- 2 tbsp maple

- 1 ½ tsp salt One chickpea

- serve with Persian Rice

- Garnish using chopped Italian parsley

- Garnish with pomegranate seeds

- 1–1 ½ lb chicken thighs

- 3 cups yellow onion, diced

- 1/4 cup pomegranate molasses

Preparation:

1. Roast the walnuts over medium flame. Blend the roasted walnuts. Cook chicken in a Dutch oven in heated oil. Set aside. Fry onions in heated oil for five minutes.

2. Stir in garlic and sauté for five minutes. Mix cinnamon, nutmeg, cumin, zest, and turmeric and sauté for a minute.

3. Pour in stock, chicken, syrup, molasses, walnuts, salt, and simmer for 45 minutes. Add the chickpeas and boil it for 15 minutes.

Roasted Chicken and White Bean Medley

Prep Time: 20 min

Cook Time: 60 min

Serve: 4

Ingredients:

- Eight teaspoons Dijon mustard

- Eight skin-on bone-in chicken thighs (about 2 pounds)

- Two tablespoons olive oil

- Two tablespoons coarsely chopped fresh parsley

- Two tablespoons capers with brine

- 2 (15-ounce) cans white beans, drained and rinsed

- 1/2 teaspoon freshly ground black pepper

- One large lemon, thinly sliced, seeds removed

- 1 1/2 teaspoons kosher salt

Preparation:

1. Preheat oven to 425 °F. In a baking dish, toss capers, beans & distribute them on the tray.

2. Spread mustard in beans & capers on the skin of every chicken. Put lemon pieces all around & beneath chicken & add insufficient water. Spice the dish with black pepper & sea salt & spray chicken with oil.

3. Insert the instant-read thermometer in chicken and roast it until skin becomes brown for thirty-five minutes

4. Switch the pan on the lower rack of the oven if the chicken starts to smoke while finishing the frying process.

5. Place prepared chicken in a bowl and decorate it with slices of lemon, capers, & beans. Put chicken sauce across the bowl and sprinkle it with parsley.

South-Western Chicken Salad

Prep Time: 10 min

Cook Time: 0 min

Serve: 6

Ingredients:

- 1 cup crushed tortilla chips
- 1 and 1/2 cups black beans
- 1 and 1/2 cups corn
- One avocado, diced
- One teaspoon minced garlic
- 1/2 cup plain Greek yogurt (use nonfat)
- 1/2 jalapeño, finely diced
- 1/2 red onion, diced
- Two teaspoons apple cider vinegar
- Two heaping teaspoons taco seasoning (use mild)
- Two teaspoons honey

- Two tomatoes, diced

- 3 Tablespoons extra virgin olive oil

- 3/4 cup shredded cheddar cheese

- 6 cups chopped romaine lettuce

- 6 cups cubed cooked chicken*

Dressing:

- handful chopped cilantro

- juice of 1 lime

- salt, to taste and if needed

Preparation:

Add all the ingredients to the bowl and mix them except salt Pour the dressing over the salad and toss it. Serve it cold.

The best turkey chili ever

Prep Time: 15 min

Cook Time: 60 min

Serve: 1

Ingredients:

- Three cloves of garlic, minced

- Two teaspoons hot sauce

- Two tablespoons olive oil

- Two tablespoons chili powder

- 2 pounds lean ground turkey

- 2 cups chicken or vegetable broth

- 1/2 teaspoon cayenne pepper (optional)

- One yellow pepper, chopped

- One yellow bell pepper, chopped

- One teaspoon garlic powder

- One teaspoon dried oregano

- One teaspoon dried basil

- One tablespoon brown sugar

- One sweet onion, finely chopped

- One red bell pepper, chopped

- 1/2 teaspoon sea salt

- 28oz crushed tomatoes

- 28oz black beans, drained

- 15oz petite diced tomatoes

- 15oz of kidney or pinto beans

Toppings: Sour cream, green onions, limes, shredded cheddar cheese

Preparation:

1. Heat the olive oil in a heavy bottom pot over medium-high & heat it till it shimmers. Add-In the ground turkey & simmer for 9 minutes, smashing it individually with a wooden spoon's help until it turned brown.

2. Add more olive oil if needed & whisk in onions & garlic.

3. Cook for 3 minutes before soften & fragrant.

4. Add peppers & again cook for three more minutes. Place the fried turkey in the pot again & then add the remaining ingredients to it. Stir & bring to a boil once combined.

5. Simmer this till the chili cooked completely 7 left it uncovered for 45 to 65 minutes until it becomes dense.

Warm Chicken Pasta Salad

Prep Time: 5 min

Cook Time: 18 min

Serve: 3

Ingredients:

- 375g dried rigatoni pasta

- 500g Lilydale Free Range Chicken Breast, trimmed

- One medium brown onion, thinly sliced

- One garlic clove, crushed

- 200g semi-dried tomatoes, drained, chopped

- 300ml pure cream

- 50g baby rocket

- 1/2 teaspoon dried chili flakes

- 1/4 cup olive oil

Preparation:

1. Take frypan and cook pasta until it becomes soft to follow the pasta packet's instructions and drain the remaining water. Along with that, heat 1 tbsp. Oil in a pan and add chicken to it.

2. Cook every side until it is completely cooked. Remove frypan from the stove, cover it & set it aside for 6 minutes. Take the remaining oil in a frypan, heat it over medium heat, and then add the onion. Cook for 4 to 6 minutes, mix frequently, or till the onion has softened. Onions, Garlic, & chili are added. Cook for 1 minute or till the smell is floral.

3. Now add cream, then cook for 4 to 6 minutes, or till the mixture thickens, stirring regularly.

4. Put a bowl of spaghetti, chicken, and rocket. Add the onions mixture. To combine, toss. Just serve.

Cinnamon Buckwheat Bowls

Prep Time: 5 min

Cook Time: 15 min

Serve: 1

Ingredients:

- ½ cup buckwheat groats, rinsed
- ½ cup almond milk or milk of choice
- ½ teaspoon cinnamon
- ½ cup water
- ½ teaspoon vanilla
- Honey to serve
- Sliced fruit to serve

Preparation:

1. In a small saucepan, add washed buckwheat grains, water, almond milk, cinnamon, and vanilla. Boil and then

simmer and cover with a lid. Cook over low heat for 10 minutes.

2. Turn off the heat and steam, covered, for an additional 5 minutes.

3. Pour with a fork and divide it into a bowl. Fill with fruit slices, sprinkle more milk and chopped honey if desired.

Sirtfood Salmon Salad

Prep Time: 10 min

Cook Time: 0 min

Serve: 1

Ingredients:

- 1 cup rocket
- oz. chicory leaves
- 1 tablespoon capers
- oz. avocado, peeled, stoned and sliced
- oz. smoked salmon slices
- 1/8 cup walnuts, chopped
- 1 large medjool date, pitted and chopped
- Juice of ¼ lemon
- 1 tablespoon extra-virgin olive oil
- 3/8 cup parsley, chopped

- ½ oz. celery leaves

- ¼ cup red onion, sliced

Preparation:

1. Place the salad leaves in a big bowl.

2. Mix all the other ingredients and serve on the leaves.

Arugula, Egg, and Charred Asparagus Salad

Prep Time: 5 min

Cook Time: 15 min

Serve: 4

Ingredients:

- oz. medium asparagus, trimmed

- ½ teaspoon black pepper, divided large eggs in shells

- 1 tablespoon fresh lemon juice

- oz. baby arugula

- 1 tablespoon extra-virgin olive oil

- 1 tablespoon water

- ¼ cup plain whole-milk Greek yogurt

- 1 teaspoon kosher salt, divided

Preparation:

1. Preheat broiler to high. Bring a small saucepan filled with water to a boil. Carefully add eggs. Cook for 8 minutes. Place eggs in a bowl filled with ice water and let stand for 2 minutes. Peel eggs, cut into quarters and sprinkle with ¼ teaspoon salt and 1/8 teaspoon pepper.

2. Combine olive oil, ¼ teaspoon salt, ¼ teaspoon pepper, and asparagus on a baking sheet. Spread in a single layer in pan. Boil for 3 minutes or until lightly charred. Remove asparagus mixture from the pan and cut into 2 inch pieces.

3. Combine remaining ¼ teaspoon salt, remaining 1/8 teaspoon pepper, yogurt, juice, and 1 tablespoon water in a medium bowl, stirring with a whisk. Add arugula and toss.

4. Arrange arugula mixture on a platter. Top with asparagus mixture and eggs. Enjoy!

Spring Vegetable and Quinoa Salad with Bacon

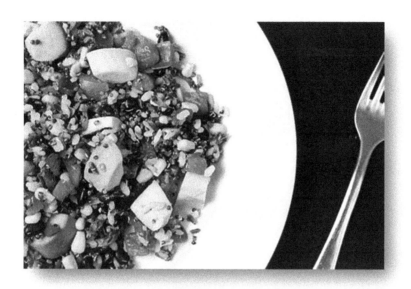

Prep Time: 5 min

Cook Time: 10 min

Serve: 4

Ingredients:

- 1 ¾ cups ginger-coconut quinoa

- cups fresh asparagus, cut diagonally into 1 inch pieces

- center-cut bacon slices, chopped

- 1 tablespoon unsalted butter

- tablespoons cider vinegar

- ½ cup frozen green peas

- teaspoons whole-grain

- Dijon mustard oz. baby spinach

- tablespoons sliced almonds, toasted

- 1 teaspoon black pepper

- 1 tablespoon fresh thyme leaves

- 1 tablespoon chopped fresh tarragon

- ½ cup chopped fresh flat-leaf parsley

Preparation:

1. Boil a large pot filled with water. Add asparagus and peas. Boil for 2 minutes, then drain. Plunge into a bowl of ice water and drain.

2. Cook the bacon in a large saucepan over medium-high heat, stirring occasionally. Remove bacon from the pan with a slotted spoon. Set aside.

3. Add vinegar, butter, and Dijon mustard to drippings in the pan, stirring with a whisk until butter melts. Add quinoa and pepper to the pan—cook for 1 minute.

4. Place quinoa mixture in a medium bowl. Add asparagus mixture, parsley, tarragon, thyme, and spinach, tossing to combine. Divide quinoa mixture among 4 plates; sprinkle evenly with reserved bacon and almonds.

Golden Chicory in Prosciutto Wraps

Prep Time: 20 min

Cook Time: 55 min

Serve: 1

Ingredients:

- heads of chicory

- slices prosciutto or Serrano ham

- 75 ml vegetable stock or white wine

- tablespoons butter

- tablespoons Dijon mustard

- ¼ cup whipping cream thyme sprigs

- slices, about 2 oz. melting cheese (cheddar is great)

- Sauté potatoes and green salad to serve

Preparation:

1. Preheat oven to 350 °F. Cut a cross from the base in the middle of the end of each chicory head. Fill the butter in the grooves, and then place the slices of Serrano ham in pairs on the work surface, overlapping them slightly. Paint the ham with mustard and spread the radish on top.

2. Pull each radish head away from you, comfortably wrapping it in the ham. Place the radish wrapped in an oven or small skillet, pour over the vegetable stock or white wine on top with the thyme sprigs. Cover the plate with loose foil and bake for 30-40 minutes until the radish is soft.

3. Unlock the plate, place the cheese slices on the chicory and bake, keep uncovered for another 6-8 minutes, until the cheese is melted and browned.

4. The radish is now ready to serve. For an extra touch, remove the chicory, place the pan on medium heat and boil

the juices with the cream for 4-5 minutes until they are rich and syrupy. Pour the sauce over the radish. Serve with sautéed potatoes and salad.

Vegetable Cabbage Soup

Prep Time: 5 min

Cook Time: 15 min

Serve: 6

Ingredients:

- ½ large head cabbage, chopped

- 1 large onion, chopped

- stalks celery, minced carrots, chopped

- tablespoons extra virgin olive oil cloves

- garlic, minced

- ½ teaspoon chili powder

- 1 can white beans, draineed and rinsed

- 1 can chopped fire-roasted tomatoes

- 1 pinch red pepper flakes

- 1 teaspoon thyme leaves

- cups low-sodium vegetable broth

- tablespoons freshly of chopped parsley, and more for garnish
- Kosher salt
- Freshly ground black pepper cups water

Preparation:

1. In a large pot over medium heat, heat olive oil. Add onion, celery, and carrots, and season with salt, pepper, and chili powder. Cook, stirring often, until vegetables are soft, 5 to 6 minutes. Stir in beans, thyme, and garlic and cook until garlic is fragrant, about 30 seconds.

2. Add broth and water, and bring to a simmer.

3. Stir in tomatoes and cabbage and simmer until cabbage is wilted, about 6 minutes. Remove from heat and stir in red pepper flakes, and parsley. Season to taste with salt and pepper. Garnish with more parsley, if desired. Enjoy!

Fresh Herb Frittata

Prep Time: 10 min

Cook Time: 15 min

Serve: 6

Ingredients:

- fresh eggs
- tablespoons chopped fresh parsley
- tablespoons chopped fresh oregano
- scallions, sliced thin, using both white and green parts
- ½ cup heavy cream
- ¾ cup finely grated parmesan cheese, divided into ½ cup and 1/4 cup portions
- Salt and pepper to taste

Preparation:

1. Preheat oven to 400 °F. In a medium mixing bowl, combine eggs, parsley, scallions, oregano, ½ cup of cheese, and heavy cream. Whisk together until thoroughly combined—season with salt and pepper, to taste.

2. In a 10-inch spicy cast iron pot, heat about 1 tablespoon of olive oil over medium heat. Add the egg mixture and cook for about 5 minutes or until the edges start to come out.

3. Sprinkle the remaining cup of cheese over the eggs.

4. Transfer the skillet to the oven and bake for 10-12 minutes, or until the cakes are puffy, the edges are visible and shake a little in the center.

5. Bake on low for about 30-45 seconds to brown the lid.

Herb-Roasted Olives and Tomatoes

Prep Time: 10 min

Cook Time: 20 min

Serve: 4

Ingredients:

- 1 cup Greek olives

- 1 cup garlic-stuffed olives

- cups cherry tomatoes

- 1 cup pitted ripe olives

- 1 tablespoon herbs de Provence

- tablespoons olive oil

- garlic cloves, peeled

- ¼ teaspoon pepper

Preparation:

1. Preheat oven to 425 °F. Combine cherry tomatoes, garlic-stuffed olives,

2. Greek olives, pitted ripe olives, and garlic cloves on a greased baking pan. Add oil and seasonings.

3. Toss to coat. Roast until tomatoes are softened, 15-20 minutes, stirring occasionally.

Grilled Asparagus with Caper Vinaigrette

Prep Time: 5 min

Cook Time: 10 min

Serve: 6

Ingredients:

- 1 ½ pounds asparagus spears, trimmed

- teaspoons caper, coarsely chopped

- 1 tablespoon red wine vinegar

- 1 garlic clove, minced

- tablespoons extra virgin olive oil

- ¼ cup small basil leaves

- ½ teaspoon Dijon mustard

- Cooking spray

- ½ teaspoon kosher salt, divided

- ¼ teaspoon freshly ground black pepper

Preparation:

1. Preheat grill to medium-high heat.

2. Place asparagus in a shallow dish. Add 1 tablespoon oil and ¼ teaspoon salt, tossing well to coat. Place asparagus on grill rack coated with cooking spray. Grill 4 minutes or until crisp-tender, turning after 2 minutes.

3. Combine remaining ¼ teaspoon salt, vinegar, mustard, and garlic. Stir with a whisk. Slowly pour remaining 2 tablespoons oil into vinegar mixture, stirring constantly with a whisk. Stir in capers. Arrange asparagus on a serving platter. Drizzle with vinaigrette, and sprinkle with basil.

Herby Pork with Apple & Chicory Salad

Prep Time: 5 min

Cook Time: 15 min

Serve: 4

Ingredients:

- oz. pork tenderloin, trimmed of any sinew and fat large apples, cored and sliced
- 270g pack chicory, leaves separated
- 1 tablespoon honey
- 1 tablespoon walnut oil
- 1 tablespoon chopped parsley
- 1 tablespoon chopped tarragon
- teaspoons wholegrain mustard
- Juice of 1 lemon

Preparation:

1. Preheat oven to 350°F. Grate pork with 1 teaspoon oil, 1 teaspoon mustard, and a few spices. Brown, transfer to a baking sheet and squeeze half of the herbs. Bake for 15 minutes until well cooked.

2. To make the salad, mix the lemon juice, honey, and the rest of the walnut oil and mustard. Period and add apples, radishes, and other herbs. Serve the sliced pork with the salad on the side.

Tomato Green Bean Soup

Prep Time: 15 min

Cook Time: 30 min

Serve: 4

Ingredients:

- 1 ½ cups diced fresh tomatoes

- ½ cup chopped onion

- ½ pound fresh green beans cut into 1 inch pieces

- ½ cup chopped carrots

- 1/8 cup minced fresh basil

- ½ garlic clove, minced

- ¼ teaspoon salt

- 1/8 teaspoon pepper

- 1 teaspoon butter

- cups reduced-sodium vegetable broth

Preparation:

1. In a large saucepan, sauté onion and carrots in butter for 5 minutes. Stir in the broth, green beans and garlic. Bring to a boil. Reduce heat. Cover and simmer until vegetables are tender.

2. Stir in the tomatoes, basil, salt and pepper. Cover and simmer 5 minutes longer.

9 781801 903066